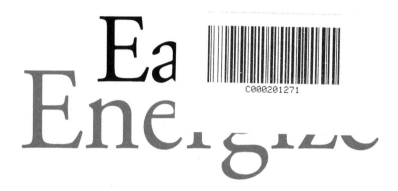

Eat Energize

Strategies and Recipes for Using the #1 Super Food for Energy

Leah E. McCullough

Praise for Leah McCullough

Leah is an expert in collaborating information needed by those whom are suffering from Fibromyalgia. If you or anyone you love has this horrendous condition, I strongly encourage you to talk to Leah!

Victoria Smith
Board Certified Holistic Practitioner,
founder of *Significant Healing Well Care Practice*

It's only been 2 days but I got up today with so much energy I vacuumed and cleaned my whole downstairs while entertaining my 6 month old!! For the first time in MANY years, I am truly hopeful that this protocol might be the one!! I can't wait until I am living out the whole book completely! So grateful for you Leah E McCullough!! And so will my whole family!!

Liz C.
St. Louis, Missouri, USA

Leah is a wonderful and caring person who really understands the health challenges people face and how to eliminate them. Her own story of recovery from fibromyalgia is inspiring and gives real hope to people with this debilitating condition.

Maria Meiners
Owner of *Delling Services*

Cover photo by Frank Fennema/Shutterstock.com

Printed in the United States of America

First Printing, 2017

ISBN 978-1-945091-28-5

Ordering Information: Special discounts are available on quantity purchases by bookstores, corporations, associations, and others. For details, contact the publisher at:

sales@braughlerbooks.com
or at 937-58-BOOKS

For questions or comments about this book, please write to:

info@braughlerbooks.com

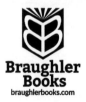

Braughler Books
braughlerbooks.com

This book was debuted at
Wise Traditions
The International Conference of
The Weston A Price Foundation
November 11, 2016
Montgomery, Alabama

A Child's Thank You Prayer

Thank You for the world so Sweet
Thank You for the food we Eat
Thank You for the birds that Sing
Thank You, God, for Everything

Acknowledgements

This book would have not been possible without the valuable knowledge that has been imparted through the Weston A. Price Foundation and its leaders and members. Weston A. Price was a dentist and researcher that looked for ways to bring the accumulated knowledge of healthy peoples to our modern world.

The leaders and members of the foundation work tirelessly to spread the word about proper nutrition for the human body. Their efforts have had a direct impact on my health and my ability to take good care of my family. For this reason and more, I am incredibly grateful.

Table of Contents

Introduction

While this book is not about fibromyalgia and chronic fatigue, per se, the strategies I used to recover from these, and then go on to have incredible energy, can be used by anyone to help get all the energy they want to help them through their busy day. **I believe energy is like money, it always helps to have more.**

The fatigue and exhaustion experienced with fibromyalgia, chronic fatigue syndrome, and ME is not a trifling matter. It can range from a feeling of "being tired all the time" to being "so tired I can't sleep." Some people are able to work, but as soon as they come home they

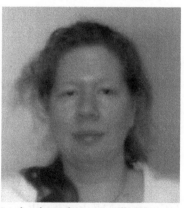

Leah when she was still sick.

need to go to bed. Others are so impaired that they just stay in bed, and over the course of a day, only have enough energy to zap something in the microwave or take a bath, not both. It takes so much energy to accomplish anything, I liken it to walking underwater, uphill, in mud. Ugh!

My experience with fibromyalgia and chronic fatigue was typical of many cases. For the last six years of my illness I was in bed 12-16 hours a day and in an incredible amount of pain. Fibromyalgia and chronic fatigue were just the tip of the iceberg: I also had major depression, anxiety, IBS (Irritable Bowel Syndrome), infertility with painful periods, migraines, PTSD, insomnia, and I was morbidly obese.

At the height of my illness I was on nine different prescription medications, three of which were just for pain, and on countless nutritional supplements. (In my book *Freedom from Fibromyalgia: 7 Steps to Complete Recovery*, I go into great detail about how I recovered from all of these conditions.)

I had no life! I lost most of my friends, I couldn't work and my family thought I was on too many prescription drugs. The isolation and loneliness was overwhelming. I was in a black pit of despair and the brain fog was so bad that I could not think my way out.

Needless to say, I am passionate about getting out this message of healing because I understand how detrimental to one's health and quality of life these diseases can be.

In this book, I am focusing on the best food sources of energy I have found. It won't "cure" fibromyalgia, chronic fatigue, or ME, but it will go a long way in helping with the symptoms of fatigue.

If you are fortunate and do not suffer with these conditions, then you will be pleasantly surprised by how much energy you will have during the day! It works even better when combined with a system of digestive healing and detoxification as described in my book, mentioned above.

The Sacred but Forgotten Food for Energy

What is this mundane food that is not an exotic berry you have never heard about from a continent you have never been?

What is this super-energy food that is available in nearly every grocery store?

Before I reveal this food I'll give you three hints to see if you can guess what it is:

1. It was considered so sacred to a traditional tribe in Africa, they used special tools so no human hands would touch it.

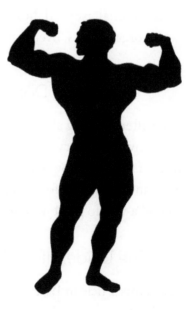

2. It is an old-school body builder supplement, from back in the 1950s.

3. This might be the give-away: your great-grand-mother probably ate it once a week.

Any guesses??

The answer is it's liver! Yes, yes it's liver! So, before you shut me out, just hold on and let me explain and I promise I will not ask you to eat liver and onions, ok?!

- Liver is one of the most nutrient-dense foods available. It is a powerhouse of nutrition and contains vitamins that are generally difficult to get in your diet such as A, D and K_2. It can even be a source of Vitamin C when consumed raw, which I will explain a little later. Stay with me please.

- The liver in traditional cultures, such as in Africa and the Native Americans, was considered sacred. Even in *The Bible*, burnt offerings included the liver and other organ meats.

- Dr. Weston A. Price (see Appendix I) in his studies of traditional, isolated, healthy peoples found that they all ate organ meats, liver being chief among them.

But I Don't Like Liver!

Even after learning about how nutritious liver is, I was still not convinced to try it. I just could not get over the strong taste of it, and I know a lot of folks feel the same way. However, after I read the following study, I was convinced to try to find a way to get it into my diet.

The Unidentified Anti-Fatigue Factor

I read this article in *Wise Traditions*, the quarterly journal of The Weston A. Price Foundation (www.WestonAPrice.org).

In it, it quotes a 1975 Prevention Magazine story about a study by Benjamin K. Ershoff, PhD, in a July 1951 article published in the *Proceedings for the Society for Experimental Biology and Medicine.*

> Ershoff divided laboratory rats into three groups. The first ate a basic diet, fortified with 11 vitamins. The second ate the same diet, along with an additional supply of vitamin B complex. The third ate the original diet, but instead of vitamin B complex received 10 percent of rations as powdered liver.
>
> "After several weeks, the animals were placed one by one into a drum of cold water from which they could not climb out. They literally were forced to sink or swim. Rats in the first group swam for an average 13.3 minutes before giving up. The second group, which had the added fortifications of B vitamins, swam for an average of 13.4 minutes. Of the last group of rats, the ones receiving liver, three swam for 63, 83 and 87 minutes. The other nine rats in this group were still swimming vigorously at the end of two hours when the test was terminated. **Something in the liver had prevented them from becoming exhausted.** [Emphasis mine.] To this day scientists have not been able to pin a label on this anti-fatigue factor."

The way I read it, the rats swam so long the scientists got tired!

After reading this long-forgotten study, I was convinced to try and find a way to add liver into my diet without suffering the taste.

Before I became pregnant I had recovered from fibromyalgia and chronic fatigue. I had what I would consider to be normal energy. When I became pregnant, my worst symptom was fatigue, not as bad as when I was sick, but still bothersome.

After the baby was born, the fatigue let up, but when the baby napped, a lot of times I did too. When he turned about 3 years old and didn't want to nap anymore, I was really sad. He didn't need a nap anymore but I did!

While the crushing fatigue was gone, I had about normal energy, but I felt like I could use some help. I read that story about the rats and I was convinced to find a way to get liver into my diet.

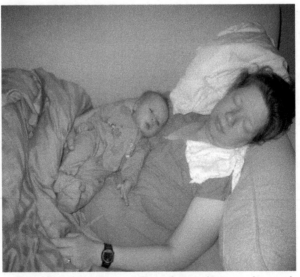

Leah with her newborn baby – notice he's awake, and mama is exhausted!

Are you convinced to learn more about giving it a try?

The 3 Easy Ways to Get the #1 Superfood into Your Diet

What needs to happen is to find a way to easily and painlessly add liver to the diet. From my research one needs to get about 1 ounce of liver a day to achieve the benefits of the anti-fatigue factor.

Listed are the 3 easy ways, and I promise liver and onions are not one of them. The ways are listed from hardest to easiest, but none of them are all that difficult.

1. Add ground up liver to any ground meat recipe that has a fair amount of spices such as spaghetti sauce or chili. The ratio so you won't taste it is 2:1. So for example, use two pounds ground meat to one pound liver. (See the recipes section.)

2. Make your own liver "pills" by taking fresh liver and cutting it up into little pieces, freezing them, and then taking a few of them every day. I get the best results from my homemade liver "pills" and because they are raw, I also benefit from Vitamin C. The main drawback is that these can be a hassle to make. (Detailed instructions on in the next section.)

3. This last way I use when I'm traveling, and I encourage people who are just starting with liver to use this way and

it is to take the old-school body building supplement, desiccated (or freeze dried) liver tablets or capsules.

You can find the old-school tablets at most health food stores. However, I have only found one brand of capsules that are minimally processed, made from grass-fed beef and are not defatted. They are available at www.RipplesHealth-Shop.com. Use coupon code ENERGY and receive a 10% discount.

When I began to supplement with liver this is how I started: first with the tablets, then the meals, and then the fresh, homemade liver "pills."

Now, I make a stew about once a week with the liver added and eat that a few times over the week. I take my homemade liver "pills" daily. And when I travel, I use the desiccated liver capsules. I use all three methods to get liver into my diet.

Note: I used to live in Germany and really enjoyed eating calf's liver pâté. It was served on buttered rolls. Since my return, I have not found any commercially prepared liver pâtés that do not have problematic ingredients in them such as MSG and sugar.

That being said, I have recently discovered the brand Trois Petits Cochons, French for Three Little Pigs, (www.3Pigs.com). I haven't done a ton of research on this brand, but the flavors are incredible and I believe them to be a good product, if you enjoy the taste of liver.

Another source of organ meats, especially if you enjoy the flavor is US Wellness Meats (www.GrassLandBeef.com). They carry liverwurst, head cheese, beef braunschweiger, and chicken braunschweiger. This company uses organic and/or pasture-raised animals, and doesn't use problematic ingredients such as MSG, etc.

Outside of the US, pâté is commonly served daily as an appetizer. If you can find an organic, pasture-raised pâté that has great ingredients, it would be a wonderful addition to your diet!

Toxins and Liver

Some people are afraid to eat liver for fear of ingesting toxins.

This is definitely a valid concern, but mostly with conventionally raised animals. Since the liver is the organ of detoxification, it makes sense that a lot of toxins would be stored there, waiting to be processed.

However, the liver is also the vitamin factory of the body and loaded with nutrition. If you buy livers from organic (and preferably pasture-raised/grass-fed) animals, the toxic load should be low and the nutrition high.

The nutrition will enhance your own liver's processing, making it more efficient at getting the toxins out of your body. **It is worth it to source high-quality food.**

Results!

Randi's 10 Mile Bike Ride to See the Pope

Before I get to my results, I want to tell you about a member of my community's results.

This is an example of adding liver and doing The Healing Cleanse (see Bonus at the end of this book).

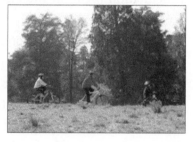

I was doing an appearance in the Washington DC area the summer before the Pope made his historic visit in 2015. A woman in the audience was a high-powered attorney with a national company you have probably heard the name of. She had a diagnosis of fibromyalgia. She sent me a very long letter about what she was not able to do before The Healing Cleanse (see Bonus) and adding liver, such as hike with her teenage daughter, who is very athletic and is a competitive swimmer.

She told me that after the talk, she immediately went to a health food store and bought liver tablets and started using them right away. After about six weeks of using the liver and doing The Healing Cleanse, she was able to ride her bicycle 10 miles over big hills to go see the Pope when he came to DC that year. She said she even had energy afterwards and her teenage daughter was worn out. This is amazing!

Leah's Results

At first I started with tablets from the health food store and I didn't really see a difference. When I started to consume the raw liver "pills" I had the best results and I noticed a big difference in only 3 days!

Now I get up between 4 and 6 am and I go all day until about 8 pm and bed at 9. I sleep very well. I might take a meditation break in the afternoon, but I certainly don't need a nap!

For me, this was the difference between 100% and 110% recovery! I now had enough energy to start a running program and I completed the Air Force Half Marathon. More importantly, I can keep up with my little boy!! His favorite thing these days is racing and he is always challenging me to run and race with him, which I love doing.

I believe one of the reasons I got such quick and positive results was because my gut had already been in healing mode for a long time and I have also continued to detoxify, while avoiding adding toxins to my body.

In my book *Freedom from Fibromyalgia: 7 Steps to Complete Recovery*, I go in depth about easy detoxification, liver, and other healing foods. The book is about one-third nutrition with lots of recipes. The book gives strategies and recipes for bulk cooking and getting nourishment even if you are too sick or too tired to cook.

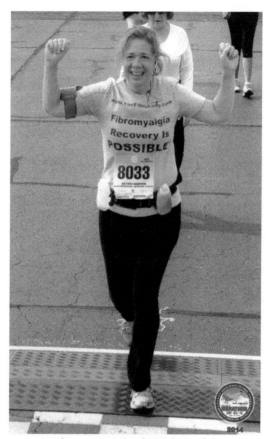

Leah crossing the finish line of the
US Air Force Half Marathon.

Instructions for Making Liver "Pills"

You will need the following:

- About 8-16 ounces, partially thawed liver from one of the following organic, grass-fed sources: beef, calf, venison, lamb or sheep (do not use poultry or pork for the raw pills)
- A cookie sheet with the raised sides that will fit in your freezer (I use a quarter-size cookie sheet)
- Wax or parchment paper
- Sharp knife
- Cutting board
- Freezer bags
- Optional ¼ cup ground cinnamon

Method:

Insure that the liver has been frozen for at least fourteen days to kill off any parasites. Let it sit out until it is partially thawed.

You will want to cut it into tiny pieces, about the size of "baby" aspirin. I like to make thin slices, then slice and dice the individual slices.

Put the pieces on a parchment-lined cookie sheet making sure they are not touching each other. Place in the freezer and leave for at least two hours or until the pieces are completely frozen. Remove cookie sheet from the freezer and immediately put the "pills" in a marked freezer bag. Store the bag in the freezer.

If the liver gets too thawed it will become slippery and difficult to cut. Put the liver back into the freezer for a short time to harden it up.

Optional: I have a friend who dredges the "pills" in ground cinnamon before putting them on the cookie sheet and she says she doesn't taste the liver at all. She says they have a lovely, cinnamon-y taste. This is a great way to get diabetes-fighting cinnamon in your diet without sugar!

How I Use the Liver "Pills"

From my research, one needs one ounce of liver a day to benefit from the anti-fatigue factor. Once a day, in the morning when I take my other supplements, I take about four of the liver "pills" (equivalent to one ounce).

They are still frozen and I really don't taste them much at all. I take them with liquid, just like a pill, but I don't chew them. In my case, within about three days I could sense a big improvement in my energy levels! (Your mileage may vary.)

Instructions for Using Desiccated Liver Capsules

Perfect Desiccated Liver

This product is made from grass-fed cow liver that has not been treated with antibiotics, hormones or pesticides. It is the only liver capsules we have found to not be defatted, just dehydrated liver put into capsules.

Loading Amount: Take 3 to 4 capsules twice a day for 30 days.

Maintenance Amount: Take 4 capsules once a day.

Pregnancy, preconception or breastfeeding: Take 3 to 4 capsules twice a day

Loading and Maintenance Amounts Explained

When starting a new supplementation regimen, some formulations have a "loading" amount, and then a maintenance amount of product to take.

In very general terms, usually the loading amount is 3 times the maintenance amount for 30 days. It is important to talk with a qualified health care practitioner as it does not apply to every situation or product.

Eat to Energize
Recipes

What Kind of Liver to Use

In my kitchen, I don't use just any kind of liver in these "hide-the-liver" recipes. Most of the time, because of its milder flavor, I use chicken liver. I save the beef, venison and lamb livers for my raw liver "pills" because they can be safely eaten without being cooked.

For poultry and pork, I cook the livers, because even though I generally buy these meats directly from organic, pasture-raised sources, I still am not comfortable eating them raw.

Often I buy a side of pork in the fall. Using pork livers with the ground pork is a great way to utilize this resource.

Main Meat of Recipe	Type of Liver to Use
Ground Beef	Chicken
Ground Lamb	Chicken or Lamb
Ground Pork	Pork
Ground Venison	Chicken or Venison

Why not other poultry? Generally, the turkey livers are sold with the entire turkey in the giblets packet. I have never seen a container of turkey livers available for sale. Because of the easy availability now of grass-fed, organic ground beef, I do not find myself purchasing ground turkey or chicken much at all.

The same goes for duck and goose. The duck and goose livers are used for a fancy and expensive type of pâté you may have heard of, *foie gras*.

What about other types of meat such as goat and fish? I do not routinely come across goat meat, and when I do, it usually just a small amount, like a roast (which when cooked slowly, is very tasty).

For fish, I'm going to leave that to another expert. I am from the Midwest of the United States and my expertise with cooking seafood is pathetically limited and beyond the scope of this book.

Type of Liver	Cooked or Raw
Chicken or another Poultry	Cooked Only
Beef	Raw, but can be cooked
Venison	Raw, but can be cooked
Pork	Cooked Only

Guidelines for Creating Your Own Recipes

In the following recipes, I generally use a ratio of 2:1. Two parts of the ground meat to one part of the livers. Since livers often come in a one pound container, often I use two pounds of the ground meat.

The other factor to hide the flavor of the liver is to have a fair amount of spices. Plain ground beef does not cover the taste of chicken liver, so I don't use this method in hamburgers, for example.

Additionally, I use ground meat because I can hide the texture of the livers very easily. In almost every recipe I cook the livers in a separate pan and then whiz them around in the food processor. If the livers are very soft, they can just be mashed with a potato masher right there in the pan while they are cooking.

This method also works for hiding other organ meats, such as hearts. Organ meats in general are powerhouses of nutrition, but the flavors can be very strong. To start I would suggest experimenting with half chicken livers and half chicken hearts. Let your imagination and ingenuity go from there!

Nourishing

These recipes are exceedingly nourishing, not only because of the organ meats, but because of the other ingredients as well.

These recipes utilize homemade stocks or broths, lots of luscious fats, and even cultured foods. Dr. Weston A. Price, (see Appendix I, The Discovery of the Perfect Human Diet), in his trips all over the world, noticed people everywhere had cooked broths, soups and stews. For multitudes of generations, people have made these dishes as an economic and nutritious way to utilize every part of the animal, obtain important nutrients, as well as fill their bellies.

In the book *Nourishing Traditions* by Sally Fallon and Mary Enig, the importance of these ingredients is explained in depth. They also explain how to bring the dietary principles of Dr. Price's healthy, "primitive" people into our modern lives.

These types of recipes have stood the test of time precisely because people have intuitively felt nourished and satisfied when eating them. Who doesn't love a bowl of chili on a crisp autumn day?!

Ingredients

Whenever possible, all animal products used in your kitchen should come from organic, pasture-raised/grass-fed sources, including lard. Except for salt, all the other ingredients should be organic. Salt should be unrefined sea salt, such as Celtic or Himalayan brands. All spices should be non-irradiated, such as Frontier brand.

Any water used should be filtered, and it is important to be free of the fluoride. Berkey brand water filters, with the fluoride filter, is an easy an economical solution to this common problem.

Kitchen Equipment

To make most of the recipes you will need the following equipment:

- A large Dutch oven pot (stainless steel or enamel over cast iron)
- 10 inch stainless steel frying pan
- A food processor

- Other basic kitchen equipment such as a knife, cutting board, etc.

If you are new to cooking for yourself, you are likely to not have decent cookware. Cheap aluminum and chipped non-stick cookware are not only frustrating to work with but are also toxic.

If you have a limited budget, then I suggest getting some good quality cookware at estate sales or even stores like Goodwill. If you have a little more room in your budget, you will get the most value from your dollar if you buy a set of pots and pans rather than individual pieces.

My current set of stainless steel pots and pans I got on HSN (Home Shopping Network) when they were having a big anniversary sale for Wolfgang Puck. I really love the quality and function, especially the glass lids so I can see what's going on without lifting the lid.

My suggestion is to purchase the best quality kitchen equipment you can afford or to even ask for pieces as gifts. People love to buy cookware as gifts, so you can let them know exactly what you would like. (I received a 7 Quart Le Cruset Dutch oven for Christmas one year and I love it!)

Storage

Admittedly, these recipes make a large amount of food. **You will find yourself blessed with nourishing meals that get better the next day!**

Because of the nature of most of the recipes in this book, they store very well. Normally I fill leftovers in a 1 quart glass Mason jar. I fill the jar to about the 3 ½ cup mark, especially if I'm going to freeze it.

Because of the amount of fat in these recipes, they kind of "seal" the food. I have been able to keep a jar of stew for many weeks in the refrigerator. However, to be safe, use refrigerated leftovers within a week, and frozen ones within six months.

If I use a starch in the recipe, such as cubed butternut squash, I layer this in the jar first, then pour the stew over it. This makes a ready-made, two or three-person meal.

Freezing: If you do freeze the jars, be sure to let them cool in the refrigerator overnight before placing them in the freezer. Only fill to the 3 ½ cup mark to give head room. Make sure you label the jar – everything looks the same when it's frozen!

To thaw: I place the frozen jar in sink full of cold water. Within about thirty minutes, the contents of the jar are usually thawed enough to work out with a wooden spoon. Otherwise, the jars can be thawed out in the refrigerator over a period of two or three days.

Stretch Your Leftovers Even Further!

What can be done with these stew recipes when you have leftovers, but not enough for a meal? Simple - make soup!

In a pot, combine the leftover stew with about 2 to 4 cups of either chicken or beef stock (I love beef broth for soups!). Check the spices to see if they are to your taste, such as adding more salt.

This is enough for an appetizer-size of soup for the entire family. The soup goes great with a salad or sandwich. AND it freezes well, to boot. All that, plus this is a great way to incorporate more stock/broth into your diet.

Energizing Chili

Serves 12

This nutrient-dense recipe makes a mild chili that is interesting for adults but most children will also like it. You can spice it up with the addition of garnishes at the table. If you want to it be low-carb, omit the beans. This recipe is also suitable for the GAPS diet.

This is an example of how I do batch cooking. Using three pounds of meat really makes a lot of food, so it is worth the effort to cook this making several meals.

For the Beans:
1 cup dry white beans
1 tablespoon Apple Cider Vinegar, lemon juice, or whey
Warm filtered water
4 cloves garlic, mashed

For the Chili:
2 tablespoons lard - separated
1 lb. chicken livers
2 lbs. ground beef

2 onions, chopped

3 tablespoons chili powder

1 tablespoon oregano

6 cloves garlic, crushed and minced

1 teaspoon red pepper sauce

2 cups beef broth/stock

1 tablespoon ground cumin

1 ½ teaspoons unrefined sea salt

1 tablespoon cocoa powder

1 cup dry red wine

2 large cans diced tomatoes

1 can tomato paste

To prepare the white beans:

A day or two ahead of when you plan on eating the chili, prepare the beans. First rinse off the beans in a colander. Put the beans in a large bowl, preferably glass, but you can also use high-quality stainless steel. There needs to be enough room in the bowl for the beans to expand at least twice their current size. Add the warm water to just cover the beans by about 2 inches. Add the acid (apple cider vinegar, lemon juice or whey) and stir. Cover to keep bugs out and let sit on the counter overnight and up to 24 hours.

After they have soaked rinse them again in the colander. Put the beans in a stock pot and add fresh filtered water to cover the beans by about two inches. Bring to a boil and skim off the foam. Add the garlic. (Do not add salt, as this can make the beans tough.) Cook for 4 hours until they are tender.

To use in recipes, drain and then add to the pot of soup, stew or chili.

I make a large quantity of beans at a time. After they are cooked I store them in 2 cup portions in the freezer to add to soups, stews and chili.

To prepare the chili:

Heat a large pot up over medium-high heat. Add 1 table-spoon lard and melt until hot. Add the ground beef and onions. Add all the spices. Cook until browned.

While the ground beef mixture is cooking, in a separate frying pan start to cook the chicken livers. Heat up the frying pan on medium-high heat. Add the remaining 1 tablespoon lard and let it melt and get hot. Add the livers (you don't have to dry them off or do anything special with them). Sprinkle with salt and pepper. Turn down the heat to medium, and later medium-low. The livers may splatter if they are cooked at too high a heat.

When the livers are browned through turn off the heat and take the frying pan over to the food processor. Put all the contents of the frying pan into the work bowl of the food processor. Put the pan back on the stove. Pulse the food processor about 7-10 times so that the livers are the consistency of ground meat. Add the livers to the ground beef mixture.

Turn the heat back on the frying pan used for the livers. Add about half the wine to the pan and deglaze it, scraping up all the cooked bits off the bottom of the pan. Add the deglazed wine and the rest of the wine to the ground meat mixture. Cook until almost all the liquid disappears.

Add the garlic, red pepper sauce, diced tomatoes, tomato paste and beef stock. Stir to combine. Add the beans at this point if you are using them. Bring to a simmer for a minimum of 20 minutes.

This recipe freezes well and is even better the next day.

Optional garnishes:

Chopped, fresh cilantro

Hot Sauce

Shredded cheese

Sour Cream

Diced Avocado

Fermented Salsa

Organic Tortilla Chips

. . . .

Energizing Beef Stroganoff

Serves 12

This is a completely different spice palate than the Energizing Chili.

Ingredients:

2 lbs. ground beef

1 lb. chicken liver/hearts

4 tablespoons oil (butter, lard, coconut oil, etc.)

2 or 3 cups beef broth/stock

1 can tomato paste

2 teaspoons salt

2 cloves garlic

2 lbs. (packages) mushrooms, sliced

2 medium onions, chopped

2 cups sour cream or plain yogurt

Method:

Heat a large pot up over medium-high heat. Add 1 tablespoon lard and melt until hot. Add the ground beef, onions, garlic, salt and mushrooms. Cook until browned.

While the ground beef mixture is cooking, in a separate frying pan start to cook the chicken livers. Heat up the frying pan on medium-high heat. Add the remaining 1 tablespoon lard and let it melt and get hot. Add the livers (you don't have to dry them off or do anything special with them). Sprinkle with salt and pepper. Turn down the heat to medium, and later medium-low. The livers may splatter if they are cooked at too high a heat.

When the livers are browned through turn off the heat and take the frying pan over to the food processor. Put all the contents of the frying pan into the work bowl of the food processor. Put the pan back on the stove. Pulse the food processor about 7-10 times so that the livers are the consistency of ground meat. Add the livers to the ground beef mixture.

Add tomato paste and beef stock, combine well and heat to a simmer. Let simmer covered for about fifteen minutes. Turn off heat and stir in sour cream.

Energizing Spaghetti Sauce

Serves 12

This is a very versatile sauce. Once made it can be used for a base for lasagna and even pizza sauce.

Ingredients:

2 tablespoons lard, coconut oil, or other fat of your choice, separated

2 onions, chopped

1 lb. chicken livers

2 lb. ground beef

¼ cup fresh parsley, finely chopped

6 cloves garlic, mashed and minced

2 bay leaves

2 tablespoons Italian seasoning

1 teaspoon unrefined sea salt

¼ teaspoon pepper

1 cup dry red wine

2 cups organic, grass-fed beef stock

2 small cans organic tomato sauce

2 small cans organic chopped tomatoes

1 small jar organic tomato paste

Note: It is preferable to buy cooked tomato products stored in glass rather than in cans.

Optional Ingredients:
2 carrots
2 stalks celery
2 pounds (packages) organic mushrooms
1 pound frozen, chopped spinach

Method:

Optional step: in the food processor, add the carrots and celery and process until finely minced.

Heat a large pot up over medium-high heat. Add 1 tablespoon lard and melt until hot. Add the ground beef, onions, garlic, parsley and optional mushrooms, and optional carrots and celery mixture. Cook until meat is browned.

While the ground beef mixture is cooking, in a separate frying pan start to cook the chicken livers. Heat up the frying pan on medium-high heat. Add the remaining 1 tablespoon lard and let it melt and get hot. Add the livers (you don't have to dry them off or do anything special with them). Sprinkle with salt and pepper. Turn down the heat to medium, and later medium-low. The livers may splatter if they are cooked at too high a heat.

When the livers are browned through turn off the heat and take the frying pan over to the food processor. Put all the contents of the frying pan into the work bowl of the food processor. Put the pan back on the stove. Pulse the food processor about 7-10 times so that the livers are the consistency of ground meat. Add the livers to the ground beef mixture.

Deglaze the liver pan with half of the wine, then add to the ground beef mixture.

Simultaneously add the salt, pepper, bay leaves, Italian seasoning, and wine to the ground beef mixture and simmer until most of the liquid evaporates.

Add the tomato sauce, chopped tomatoes, tomato paste, beef stock and optional spinach.

Let simmer covered for fifteen to thirty minutes. For thicker sauce, simmer uncovered to let the liquid evaporate.

Serving suggestions:

Serve over noodles, sautéed butternut squash cubes, or roasted spaghetti squash.

Generously sprinkle with grated parmesan cheese.

....

Energizing Taco Meat

Serves 6

This is a great recipe is a great example of the 2:1 ratio of meat to liver, but only using one pound of meat. You can add this meat mixture to tacos, enchiladas, burritos, or even to warm up a salad.

Ingredients:

1 tablespoon lard, coconut oil, or other fat of your choice, separated

1 lb. ground beef

½ lb. (8 ounces) chicken livers

1 tablespoon Taco Seasoning Mix (see below)

1 cup beef stock

Taco Seasoning Mix:

2 tablespoons chili powder

1 t. unrefined sea salt

½ teaspoon garlic powder

Method:

Heat a large skillet over medium-high heat. Add 1/2 table-spoon lard and melt until hot. Add the ground beef. Cook until meat is browned.

While the ground beef mixture is cooking, in a separate frying pan start to cook the chicken livers. Heat up the frying pan on medium-high heat. Add the remaining 1/2 tablespoon lard and let it melt and get hot. Add the livers (you don't have to dry them off or do anything special with them). Sprinkle with salt and pepper. Turn down the heat to medium, and later medium-low. The livers may splatter if they are cooked at too high a heat.

When the livers are browned through turn off the heat and take the frying pan over to the food processor. Put all the contents of the frying pan into the work bowl of the food processor. Put the pan back on the stove. Pulse the food processor about 7-10 times so that the livers are the consistency of ground meat. Add the livers to the ground beef mixture.

Deglaze the liver pan with half of the stock, then add to the ground beef mixture.

Add taco seasoning spice mixture and remaining beef stock to the ground beef mixture. Simmer uncovered for 10-15 minutes.

Serving Suggestions:

I prefer to have a taco salad rather than tacos, to get additional veggies. You can have all the toppings in separate dishes and everyone can make their own creations.

Toppings:

Organic Tortilla Chips

Shredded Cheese

Avocado chunks or guacamole

Fermented Salsa

Sour Cream

Hot Sauce

Chopped Cilantro

Lettuce, and other salad ingredients, such as chopped cucumbers and green onion slices

Chopped tomatoes

Bean dip

Sliced olives

Chopped onions

Olive oil or salad dressing

Energizing Shepherds Stew

Serves 12

This recipe is inspired by the English celebrity chef, Gordon Ramsey, of the television show Hell's Kitchen fame. It is based on his mum's recipe for shepherds pie filling. You can make this into shepherds pie, but I just love it as stew!

Ingredients:

4 tablespoons lard, coconut oil, or the fat of your choice, separated

2 lbs. ground lamb (or beef, or combination)

1 lb. chicken livers

2 large onions, grated or finely chopped

1 bag of frozen peas and carrot cubes

6 cloves of garlic

6 tablespoons Worcestershire sauce

1 can/bottle tomato paste

1 t. dried thyme

1 t. dried rosemary

2 cups dry red wine (optional)

2 cups chicken or beef stock

1 t. unrefined sea salt

¼ t. freshly ground black pepper

Method:

Heat a large pot up over medium-high heat. Add 2 table-spoons lard and melt until hot. Add the ground lamb, onions and garlic. Cook until meat is browned.

While the ground beef mixture is cooking, in a separate frying pan start to cook the chicken livers. Heat up the frying pan on medium-high heat. Add the remaining 2 tablespoon lard and let it melt and get hot. Add the livers (you don't have to dry them off or do anything special with them). Sprinkle with salt and pepper. Turn down the heat to medium, and later medium-low. The livers may splatter if they are cooked at too high a heat.

When the livers are browned through turn off the heat and take the frying pan over to the food processor. Put all the contents of the frying pan into the work bowl of the food processor. Put the pan back on the stove. Pulse the food processor about 7-10 times so that the livers are the consistency of ground meat. Add the livers to the ground beef mixture.

Deglaze the liver pan with half of the wine, then add to the ground lamb mixture.

Simultaneously add the salt, pepper, thyme, rosemary, tomato paste, Worcestershire sauce, and wine to the ground beef mixture and simmer until most of the liquid evaporates.

Add the stock/broth as well as the frozen peas and carrots.

Let simmer uncovered for fifteen minutes, or until desired thickness. For thicker stew, simmer uncovered to let the more of the liquid evaporate. When the desired thickness is reached, cover and let simmer for a total of 30 minutes.

Serving suggestions:

Serve with or over mashed potatoes or with sautéed butternut squash cubes. Serve with sour cream.

. . . .

Energizing Beef Meatballs

Serves 12, about 5 dozen meatballs

Admittedly, making up a large batch of meatballs can be very time-consuming. However, once made, they are extremely versatile to have on hand. They can be heated up and served on their own as part of a busy week-night supper, added to a jar of spaghetti sauce for spaghetti and meatballs, added to soups, or even used as a cocktail appetizer, with or without sauce.

Ingredients:

2 lbs. ground beef
1 lb. chicken livers
1 ½ cups finely ground almond flour
½ cup milk
1 ½ t. unrefined sea salt
½ t. pepper
1 ½ t. organic Worcestershire sauce
1 medium onion, finely chopped
2 eggs
¾ cup of fresh parsley, finely chopped

Method:

Preheat oven to 400° F.

In a food processor, add the raw chicken livers. Hit the pulse button about seven times in order to get the livers to the consistency of the ground beef, or even finer. Be careful not to liquefy them.

Mix all ingredients, except the lard, in a large mixing bowl. You may have to use your hands. Shape into sixty, 1½ inch meatballs.

Unlike a stew, once meatballs are cooked, there is no way to go back and adjust the spices, such as salt. Also, since they are raw, and there is the presence of raw chicken, they must be tested in a cooked state. Therefore, to test the seasoning of the meatballs make a few balls, cook in a frying pan with a little fat, such as lard. Taste to see if any adjustments are needed.

When the spices are to your taste, arrange the meatballs, twenty at a time, on a 9x13x2 inches tempered glass rectangular pan, such as Pyrex. Bake 20 to 25 minutes, turning once, until no longer pink inside. This recipe will make three pans of meatballs.

To Panfry:

Over medium heat, heat a large skillet. Add 1 tablespoon lard, coconut oil or your favorite fat. When melted add as many meatballs to the skillet without them touching. You will have to work in batches and you may need to add additional oil as you progress. Make sure the oil is melted and hot before you add the meatballs.

Storage

Once the meatballs are cooked they are ready to be one of the most easy and versatile energizing foods in your home!

Use a cookie sheet that will fit in your freezer (a quarter size sheet for a side-by-side, and a half size sheet for top freezer refrigerators). Place a sheet of parchment, wax, or freezer paper on the cookie sheet.

Place the meatballs on the cookie sheet, as many as will fit *without touching*. Freeze for at least three hours or better if overnight. Once frozen, put in gallon-sized freezer bags that have been labeled.

Reheating Instructions

You can reheat these meatballs directly from the freezer, or they can be thawed first.

To bake from frozen

Preheat oven to 350° F. In a shallow baking dish heat meatballs for 25-30 minutes, turning once.

Stovetop

This method works better when the meatballs are thawed. In sauce or stock, gently simmer the meatballs until hot in the center. In a frying pan, over medium heat, sauté meatballs in melted fat until hot in the center, about ten minutes.

Energizing Prussian Meatballs

Serves 12

This is an amazing recipe that I am really excited to share! You won't find anything like this in any other American cookbooks.

In the early 1990s, I was a typical American twenty-something-year-old, living in western part of the newly reunified Germany. When I would go over to my "mutti's" house, this was my favorite dish she would make.

My "mutti" explained to me that was taught to make this from her mother-in-law, who was from the former Prussian territory Konigsberg (nowadays, since the end of World War II, the Russian territory of Kaliningrad).

Ignorantly, I turned my nose up at most of the traditional food, thinking it was too fatty and therefore, fattening. I used to say German food was meat, potatoes, and a side of grease.

While the ingredients to this recipe seem kind of odd, they create a unique and satisfying dish. If a typical American young woman loved it, it must be good!

I have only made a slight few modifications from the traditional Prussian version, Konigsberg Klopse, by adding the pork liver, and substituting almond flour for day-old bread.

I want to encourage you to give this a try in your home. Let me know what you think about it!

Ingredients:

2 lbs ground pork

1 lbs pork liver or combination of liver and heart

1 cup apple cider vinegar

2 cups of water

2 medium onions, finely chopped (reserving 1 teaspoon for sauce)

10 anchovies, very finely chopped, or 1 tablespoon anchovy paste

4 eggs

2 tablespoons minced parsley

Grated rind of 2 lemons

1 teaspoon salt

½ teaspoon pepper

8 cups beef or pork stock/broth

Sauce:

1 tablespoon butter

1 teaspoon reserved onion, minced

2 tablespoons capers

4-6 tablespoons sour cream

Note: Traditionally, fresh pork meat was marinated in an acidic solution before cooking. Some speculate it was to neutralize the potential parasites. The Weston A. Price Foundation published an article in their quarterly journal, Wise Traditions, showing the effects on live blood by eating pork prepared in various ways. The article can be found at this web address: http://www.westonaprice.org/health-topics/how-does-pork-prepared-in-various-ways-affect-the-blood/ .

Method:

Optional Step: (After reading the above-mentioned Wise Traditions article, I hope you agree that this is not an optional step.) The day before you want to eat the meatballs, marinate the meat. In a food processor, add the liver and optional heart (that has been cut in slices) to the work bowl. Pulse until it is about the same consistency as the ground pork.

In a large bowl combine the ground pork and the ground liver, or liver and heart mince. Add the apple cider vinegar, and then enough filtered water to cover the meat. Work the vinegar mixture into the ground meat a little. Let sit in the refrigerator, covered, for about eight hours.

Remove about half of the meat onto a lint free kitchen towel, squeezing out as much of the marinade as possible. With about half the meat in the towel, squeeze as much water out of the meat as possible. Place the dry meat in a different, clean, large mixing bowl. Repeat this with the second half of the meat.

If you do not do the above-mentioned optional step, start out by adding the sliced liver and/or heart to the food processor and pulse until it is finely minced. Put the organ mince and ground pork in a large mixing bowl.

Add the remaining ingredients except for the stock and sauce ingredients. Mix well, you will probably end up using your hands. Simultaneously while you're mixing the ingredients, in a large Dutch oven pot, bring to a simmer the 8 cups of stock.

Unlike a stew, once meatballs are cooked, there is no way to go back and adjust the spices, such as salt. Also, since they are raw, and there is the presence of raw pork, they must be tested in a cooked state. Therefore, to test the seasoning of the meatballs make a ball, cook in a small pot of broth (about one cup). Taste to see if any adjustments are needed.

Shape the mixture into balls that are 2 1/2 inches in diameter (about the size of golf ball). You are welcome to make them smaller, just adjust your cooking time down.

Working in small batches, while maintaining hot but not boiling broth, carefully cook the meatballs in the broth for approximately 15 minutes, turning at least once. Boiling broth can cause the meatballs to fall apart. As the meatballs are cooked set them aside and keep warm.

After the meatballs are finished, it's time to work on the sauce. Add all the sauce ingredients except the sour cream, to the broth pot and simmer until it reduces and becomes thicker. Turn down the heat and stir in the sour cream. Once combined add the meatballs back into warm up, or if you have kept them warm in a covered dish in the oven, serve them separately with the sauce on top.

Serving suggestions

Traditionally, these meatballs and sauce are served with boiled, cubed potatoes or with the German noodle, spaetzle. Cooked red cabbage is also a nice side.

Storage

You can store the meatballs individually like with the beef meatballs recipe, or they can be stored with the sauce, which is probably easier.

For individual meatball storage: Use a cookie sheet that will fit in your freezer (a quarter size sheet for a side-by-side, and a half size sheet for top freezer refrigerators). Place a sheet of parchment, wax, or freezer paper on the cookie sheet.

Place the meatballs on the cookie sheet, as many as will fit *without touching*. Freeze for at least three hours or better if overnight. Once frozen, put in gallon-sized freezer bags that have been labeled.

Reheating Instructions

You can reheat these meatballs directly from the freezer, or they can be thawed first.

To bake from frozen:

Preheat oven to 350° F. In a shallow baking dish heat meatballs for 25-30 minutes, turning once.

Stovetop:

This method works better when the meatballs are thawed. In sauce or stock, gently simmer the meatballs until hot in the center. In a frying pan, over medium heat, sauté meatballs in melted fat until hot in the center, about ten minutes.

. . . .

Raise the Dead Chicken Broth Recipe

Makes about 5 Quarts

While this is not an "energizing" recipe, it is in an integral part of many of the recipes in this book. This is my basic recipe for some of the best-tasting broth I have ever had. I have never actually tried to raise a dead person with it, but it is so yummy and nourishing I'm confident it would work!

I make broth about once a week and I make it on a day when I will be around to monitor it, like on the weekend. I start this early in the day, usually using the carcass from the chicken from the previous night. After it is finished I often go on to make chicken soup with some of the broth, so when I prepare the veggies for this recipe, I go ahead and prepare the veggies for the soup. (If I am going to peel one carrot, it's just a moment more to peel two.) However, I have made this broth without any vegetables before, just bones, vinegar, water and salt and it comes out alright too.

Ingredients:

1 organic and/or pasture-raised chicken carcass including all soft tissues such as skin and gristle

1 set of cleaned chicken feet (optional)

5 quarts of filtered water

1 tablespoon Apple Cider Vinegar (like Bragg's) or dry white wine

2 carrots, peeled and coarsely chopped

1 celery stalk, coarsely chopped

1 onion, coarsely chopped

1 freezer bag of veggie scraps (optional)

Egg shells from organic and/or pasture raised chickens, rinsed (optional)

2 tablespoons unrefined sea salt (like Himalayan or Celtic Sea Salt)

5 black peppercorns

1 bunch of parsley, rinsed well

Method:

(Optional Step) On a cutting board, take the large bones of the chicken, such as leg and thigh, and with a meat hammer, break in half. This will release the nutrients inside the bone marrow.

If the chicken carcass is raw, then there is usually a lot of meat on the back that can be cooked and taken off during the process of making broth. This meat is usually the perfect amount for a pot of chicken soup!

If your carcass is frozen, that is fine and you can begin as normal. In a large stock pot, preferably stainless steel, place chicken carcass, chicken feet (optional), egg shells (optional), water and vinegar (or wine), and veggies together and let sit for 30 minutes. This will give the vinegar time to release the nutrients from the carcass. (I use an eight-quart stock pot for the recipe or a twenty-quart stock pot if I triple the recipe.)

Add the salt and peppercorns and bring to an almost boil, a simmer.

Skim the foam off the top. (I do this with a large, long-handled stainless spoon and put into a bowl nearby. I skim several times over the next 30 minutes or so.) Be careful not to pick up the veggies or peppercorns, or just rinse them off and return them to the pot. Also, be careful not to let the pot come to a rolling boil as this will dissipate the foam and could dry out any meat that you are cooking.

At this point if you are using a raw carcass check the back to see if it is cooked through. If it looks like it is, remove it and set it aside to cool. After it has cooled pick the meat off and return the skin and bones to the pot. Save the meat for soups or stews. Between the neck and back of a large chicken, I can get almost a cup of meat.

If you are using a **whole chicken**, watch carefully for the meat to cook through in about 1 ½ hours of simmer time. Don't let the water get to a boil, it will dry the meat out. Also, the breast meat will cook faster, so you might want to remove the bird, let cool, take off the breasts and wings, then return to let the legs and thighs cook some more. Remove the meat and add the soft tissues and bones back to the pot and continue to cook the broth.

For the last 10 minutes of cooking add the bunch of parsley.

You can cook the broth anywhere from a minimum of 3 hours to a maximum of 3 days. My family prefers the 3-hour broth the best.

Note on veggie scraps: When preparing veggies for your meals save the scraps in a gallon freezer bag to be kept in the freezer. Broccoli stalks, ends of zucchini, etc. and even fruit scraps such as apple cores can be used. They add a nice flavor to the broth and use up a great resource. You can also keep a freezer bag of chicken scraps going too and add those in at the beginning. I keep a bag in my freezer labeled "Bits for Broth."

What's the difference between broth and stock?

The easiest definition I have heard is that stock is made with specific ingredients so that it is consistently the same every time and broth is more free-form, using whatever you have in the kitchen. Therefore, I primarily make broth.

Storing the Broth

This method for storing the broth took me a while to figure out. I think it uses the least number of extra dishes and is the least-messy way I have found to do this. After the broth is finished cooking, let it cool slightly in the pot for easier handling.

I put the broth up in 1 or 2 quart, wide-mouth glass canning jars. Sometimes I also store only about 2 cups of broth in a jar, and mark it as such. I use either a quart jar or a pint jar for this. Most non-soup recipes that use stock call for 1 cup, and I double most recipes that I like and are familiar with. (Get the wide mouth jars and plastic lids will fit on the pint, 1 quart and 2 quart jars. They seal better than the metal lids and are easy to pop into the dishwasher. The plastic doesn't come into contact with the food.)

I like to mark my jars with a piece of freezer tape on the lid where I have written the contents with a Sharpie marker. Some also put the date. If you mark directly onto the lid or the side of the jar it is permanent. *Label the jars. It is difficult to identify anything that is frozen.*

Place a 4 or 8 cup glass measuring bowl with a pouring spout in the sink with an 8 inch stainless steel mesh strainer balanced on top. I pour the liquid from the stock pot into the strainer until either the bowl or strainer is full.

Optional step:

Pick through the solids, taking out any soft tissues, such as fat, skin, meat, etc. These soft tissues go into the food processor to be whizzed into "pâté." Place equal amounts of the "pâté" into the broth jars after all of it has been poured. Close the lids tightly and shake the jars to incorporate the "pâté" into the broth. These soft tissues are an excellent source of gelatin which is important for gut healing.

Remove the solids from the strainer and dispose. Take your jar and set it into the sink and then pour the broth from the measuring bowl spout into the jar(s). If you are planning on freezing the broth, only fill the jar up to about where it starts to curve in (at about the 3 cups mark on a 1 quart jar) to leave head room for expansion.

Place lids on the jars and let them cool on the counter for a while before placing them in the refrigerator. Let the jars stay in the refrigerator at least overnight before placing them in the freezer. This will help the jar from cracking. A jar of broth will keep for about a week in the refrigerator.

After the jars of broth have cooled, some people skim the fat off the top. I do not. Fat equals flavor and satiety. It is only important if you are making something that needs to be very clear or if you eat a diet that has a lot of processed foods.

To thaw a frozen jar quickly: Fill up the sink with cold water and place the jar inside for 20-40 minutes (do not submerge). The middle will still be frozen but it will be thawed enough to pour out and the frozen part will thaw quickly in a hot pot.

Quick Broth

This is the broth to make if you are too sick to make broth from scratch. It was inspired by *Nourishing Traditions* recipe, Quick Stock. Drink this in a mug several times a day.

Ingredients:

One 8 oz. package liquid chicken broth (I use Pacific Natural Foods Organic Free Range Chicken Broth, found in the natural section at the grocery store.)

1 teaspoon gelatin (I use Bernard Jensen's 100% Bovine Gelatin)

½ teaspoon Himalayan or Celtic Sea Salt

1 teaspoon organic, grass-fed butter (I use Kerry Gold Unsalted) or coconut oil

Method:

Place all ingredients in a saucepan and bring to a simmer. This yields one cup. You may need to add more salt.

· ·

Beef Broth

Makes about 5 Quarts

Beef broth or stock on its own is not particularly tasty, but what it does to soups and sauces is transcendent! I make a big batch and freeze in 2 cup portions so it's already recipe-sized to go.

Ingredients

5-6 pounds meaty beef bones, such as a soup bones, neck bones, oxtail, etc.

½ cup apple cider vinegar

5 quarts filtered water

2 stalks celery, coarsely chopped

3 carrots, coarsely chopped

2 onions, coarsely chopped

1 bunch fresh parsley

Unrefined sea salt

Method

Preheat oven to 350° F. Place all the bones in a 9x13x2 inch glass pan and sprinkle with salt. Cook the bones in the oven for 35 minutes, until browned. (This will impart love-ly color and flavor to your stock.)

Optional: Once the meat is out of the glass pan, pour one cup boiling hot water into the pan. With a wooden spoon scrape all the cooked bits from the bottom of the pan – that's flavor! Add all of the water with the cooked bits to the stock pot.

Place the meat, vinegar and all the veggies except the parsley in the stock pot and leave at room temperature for 30 minutes. Turn on heat and bring to a simmer.

Skim off foam and let cook at a low simmer for about three hours. During the last ten minutes of cooking add the parsley for flavor and minerals.

Store as mentioned in detail in the Raise the Dead Chicken Broth Recipe.

The Discovery of the Perfect Human Diet

Weston A. Price, DDS, was a dentist from Ohio that did some very interesting studies about nutrition in the 1930s and '40s. He saw that more and more of his patients were getting cavities and crowded teeth. He felt that the mouth was a mirror of the total health of the body. He hypothesized that nutrition, not genetics, was the root cause of the problems. He studied healthy, isolated peoples all over the world to see what their diets consisted of and what they had in common.

For example, one of the groups he studied were Eskimos in Canada. The Eskimos who lived in isolation, surviving only on the foods that they provided for themselves, not only had perfectly straight teeth with very low rates of cavities, but also had remarkable overall health. Then he contrasted those folks with another group of Eskimos who had a village by a road and had access to a store (full of processed foods). They had very crooked teeth, cavities, and degenerative diseases in just one generation of eating the processed foods. He saw this exact scenario played out over and over again in all the groups he studied all over the world.

One of the things Dr. Price discovered with all the groups of healthy isolated peoples is that they ate fat at a rate of over ten times what Americans ate in the 1930s. Of course, that figure would be much, much higher now.[i]

For more information about Dr. Price and how his findings fit in to our everyday lives go to the Weston A. Price Foundation at www.WestonAPrice.org. There are local chapters all over the US and the world.

Principles of Healthy Traditional Diets

- Eat whole, unprocessed foods.
- Eat beef, lamb, game, organ meats, poultry, and eggs from pasture-fed animals.
- Eat wild (not farm-raised) fish, shellfish, and fish roe from unpolluted waters.
- Eat full-fat milk products from pasture-fed cows, preferably raw and/or fermented, such as raw milk, whole yogurt, kefir, cultured butter, fresh and sour cream, and whole raw cheeses.
- Use animal fats, especially butter, liberally.
- Use traditional vegetable oils only: extra-virgin olive oil, expellerexpressed sesame oil, small amounts of expeller-expressed flax oil, and the tropical oils: coconut and palm oil.
- Eat fresh fruits and vegetables—preferably organic—in salads and soups, or lightly steamed with butter.
- Use whole grains*.[2]

*Note: If you choose to eat grains (which I do not) make sure they are organic and have been prepared by soaking, souring or sprouting to make them easier to digest. Eat them with liberal amounts of fat, such as butter, to lower their effect on your blood sugar. Also, most gluten-containing grains, modern wheat in particular, are not appropriate for almost everyone. I highly recommend the books *Wheat Belly* by Dr. William Davis and *Grain Brain* by Dr. David Perlmutter for thorough explanations.

Notes

1. Sally Fallon and Mary Enig, Eat Fat Lose Fat (New York: Hudson Street Press, 2005.)

2. Price, Weston A. MS, DDS, Nutrition and Physical Degeneration. New York: Medical Book Department of Harper and Brothers, 1939

Resources

Supplements

Ripples' Health Shop, LLC, "Your neighborhood health food store, online." Their contact info is as follows:

www.RipplesHealthShop.com, phone is 937-999-1369.

For Personal Help

Look for upcoming classes to be announced in the free newsletter "The Unconventional Traditional" by Leah E. McCullough, www.TheFibroLady.com.

Coaching programs are available from Natural Healing Expert Leah E. McCullough.

Contact her at Leah@TheFibroLady.com.

I hope you enjoyed my book *Eat to Energize: Strategies and Recipes for Using the #1 Superfood*. If you're feeling inspired and excited as I am after reading this, then I invite you to explore the holistic approach to recovery that I have developed with

Freedom from Fibromyalgia:
The Complete Recovery System

This holistic system has the breakthrough book *Freedom from Fibromyalgia: 7 Steps to Complete Recovery* in paperback and electronic editions, two guided meditation audios (Optimal Health and Restorative Sleep), the meditation transcripts, an instructional video, as well as 3 months of unlimited email coaching. Go to http://store.TheFibroLady .com to order your set today!

Please reach out to our fabulous team via the website www.TheFibroLady.com, or email at Leah@TheFibroLady. com.

We're here to help!
Yours in joyful health,
Leah

About Leah E. McCullough

Leah E. McCullough, affectionately known as **The Fibro Lady**, is the voice for fibromyalgia recovery.

Leah is America's foremost Natural Healing Expert. She teaches people around the world how to regain their optimal health and energy levels. She is a national speaker and author of the book *Freedom from Fibromyalgia: 7 Steps to Complete Recovery*. She has been interviewed on radio, television and the Internet about fibromyalgia recovery.

She currently lives with her family in the Dayton, Ohio area and recently completed the US Air Force Half Marathon.

Contact her at Leah@TheFibroLady.com.

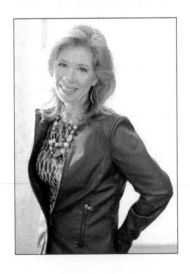

Bonus

Go to the Resources tab on www.TheFibroLady.com and select Bonus to claim your copy of The Healing Cleanse.